DATE DUE

PATERSON AND ZDERAD

Notes on Nursing Theories

SERIES EDITORS
Chris Metzger McQuiston
Private Practice

Adele A. Webb
College of Nursing, University of Akron

The purpose of this series of monographs is to provide the reader with a concise description of conceptual frameworks and theories in nursing. It is not intended to replace the primary works of nurse theorists, but to provide direction for their use. Designed for undergraduate students, these monographs will also be helpful guides for graduate students and faculty.

Due to the complexity of existing books and chapters on nursing conceptual frameworks and theories, students often have difficulty understanding and incorporating nursing theory into their practice. The concise monographs of this series include a biographical sketch of the theorist, origin of the theory, assumptions, concepts, propositions, examples for application to practice and research, glossary of terms, and a bibliography of classic works, critiques, and research. Organization of the information in this manner will facilitate student understanding and use, thereby broadening the base of nursing science.

PATERSON AND ZDERAD

Humanistic Nursing Theory

Nancy O'Connor

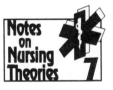

Notes on Nursing Theories 7

SAGE Publications
International Educational and Professional Publisher
Newbury Park   London   New Delhi

Copyright © 1993 by Sage Publications, Inc.

For information address:

SAGE Publications, Inc.
2455 Teller Road
Newbury Park, California 91320

SAGE Publications Ltd.
6 Bonhill Street
London EC2A 4PU
United Kingdom

SAGE Publications India Pvt. Ltd.
M-32 Market
Greater Kailash I
New Delhi 110 048 India

RT
84.5
.O35
1993

Printed in the United States of America

Library of Congress Cataloging-in-Publication Data

O'Connor, Nancy (Nancy A.)
   Paterson and Zderad: humanistic nursing theory/ Nancy O'Connor
     p.   cm.—(Notes on nursing theories; v. 7)
   Includes bibliographical references.
   ISBN 0-8039-4798-4 (cloth).—ISBN 0-8039-4489-6 (pbk.)
    1. Nursing—Philosophy. 2. Paterson, Josephine G. 3. Zderad,
Loretta T. I. Paterson, Josephine G. Humanistic nursing.
II. Zderad, Loretta T. Humanistic nursing. III. Title.
IV. Series.
RT84.5.O35 1992
610.73'01—dc20   92-32735
                                                       CIP

93 94 95 96 10 9 8 7 6 5 4 3 2 1

Sage Production Editor: Megan M. McCue

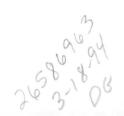

To all my significant communities,
in particular to my colleagues at
the Primary Care Nursing Service,
Detroit Receiving Hospital/
University Health Center

Contents

Foreword

The purpose of this monograph is to systematically relate humanistic nursing theory to the identified metaparadigm elements in nursing. Consequently, the humanistic nursing conceptualization with regard to person, nurse, health, and environment is recounted. Starting with (a) the individual lived experiences and lives of Drs. Josephine Paterson and Loretta Zderad, (b) the historical development of the theory, (c) the implicit assumptions, and (d) a glossary of terms, the *content* and *process* of the theory is examined.

The major phenomena of interest to creators of humanistic nursing theory are person and nurse. The theory also provides for the placement of health and environment but to a less-well-developed degree. Nursing is viewed as an authentic dialogue involving meeting, relating, and presencing in a world of people, things, time, and space. All of these concepts are explained in detail. The existential foundations of humanistic nursing include the uniqueness and sameness of each individual person along with human relating for development of potentials. The potentials, when developed by choice and authentic awareness, lead to more being and growth (health). The outcome of authentic encountering, according to Paterson and Zderad, is comfort.

Nursing occurs all at once with multifarious multiplicities, and the value of diversity with regard to setting for nursing practice is related by *inclusion* of role function and clinical focus. The weaving of the objective-subjective-intersubjective relating of the situation is suggested for phenomenological description of the lived human event of nursing. Thus the expression attributed to R. D. Laing that theory is "the articulated vision of experience" is given credence by the theorists. *Nursology* is the name given to the theorizing process. The process of nursology answers the question: How can the nurse, a subjective-objective human being, know the other and compare and complementarily synthesize the exchanges between these known others? The monograph explains the five phases of this process and the results that are transforming and inclusive for a unified insight. New creation happens as one reality from the lived situation illuminates another for additive development of general knowledge principles.

Within the monograph, the concepts of presence and dialogue are presented as examples of nursing involving doing and being in relationship. The confirming of the persons (nurse and patient) happens during "presencing." The presencing enfolds the skill or technical "doing" part of the nursing care for goal attainment. The attributes of presence are fully described within the context of the nursing situation. Dialogue as nursing is a transactive process implied as a special kind of meeting of humans for a purposeful "call and response" situation. A deep encountering happens as a result of the interchange. For future connection and direction, an example using humanistic nursing practice components is provided. The current resources and projects that involve concepts or aspects of humanistic nursing theory are listed.

Acknowledgment is given to Dr. Josephine Paterson and Dr. Loretta Zderad for the development of a theory and an explication of a phenomenological process that expresses value, commitment to, and investment in the lived experience of the patient and the nurse.

DORIS R. HINES, PHD, RN

Preface

I first became acquainted with the thinking and writing of Drs. Paterson and Zderad in 1976 upon publication of their text *Humanistic Nursing*. At that time I had the good fortune of being a registered nurse enrolled in a BSN completion program at a private college in which the educational philosophy included both a strong liberal arts thread within all majors and a pragmatic focus on preparation of baccalaureate graduates for the world of work. This institution had achieved an understanding of the appropriate blend of thinking and doing which characterizes meaningful work and sustains persons engaged in such work. Conditions were thus favorable for my first reading of *Humanistic Nursing*. I came to it as a seasoned nurse with an understanding of the practice world of nursing and as a learner receptive to new ways of thinking about my work. My readiness to learn was supported by an environment that honored both practical and conceptual ways of knowing. Thus, the essential themes in *Humanistic Nursing* made sense to me at that time in my nursing world. Reading and discussing this text with classmates and faculty was extremely influential both in making explicit our shared nursing experiences and in ushering in a glimpse of the possibility of a lifetime pursuit of nursing scholarship.

As with all enduring works, *Humanistic Nursing* both anticipates and continues to speak to important issues in contemporary nursing. For example, the value of explicating that knowledge which is unique to nursing, the creation of research methodologies which are consonant with the nursing world, the understanding of the multiple ways of knowing necessary in nursing contexts, the grounding of nursing knowledge in the nursing situation, the importance of the knower in knowledge development, and the integration of thinking, doing, and being within the nursing world, are but a few topics about which readers of the original work will gain insight. I believe that *Humanistic Nursing* will continue to be studied as a foundational work in nursing epistemology. It is my pleasure to present to the reader an abbreviated and interpreted version of this work that has been so influential in my nursing world and that continues to illuminate our collective nursing worlds. I would like to thank the series editors, Adele Webb and Chris McQuiston, for envisioning this reader friendly series of affordable text companions which can be seen as skimming the surface or as plumbing the depths of essential nursing theory texts. We in nursing continue to be ambivalent about the role of ease and pleasure in matters of nursing knowledge construction.

NANCY O'CONNOR

Biographical Sketches of the Nurse Theorists:
Josephine G. Paterson (DNS, RN)

Born: September 1, 1924, in Freeport, New York
Position: Retired from nursing, 1985; position prior to
retirement as "nursologist" at the Northport Veterans
Administration Hospital in Northport, New York
Diploma: Lenox Hill Hospital School of Nursing, New York,
August 1945
BS Nursing Education, St. John's University, Brooklyn, New
York, August 1954
MPH, Johns Hopkins School of Hygiene & Public Health, Bal-
timore, Maryland, June 1955
Specialty: mental health; fieldwork completed April 1956
DNS, Boston University, 1969; specialty: psychiatric mental health

Loretta Zderad (PhD, RN)

Born: June 7, 1925, Chicago, Illinois
Position: Retired from nursing, 1985; position prior to retire-
ment as "nursologist" at Northport Veterans Administra-
tion Hospital, Northport, New York
Diploma: St. Bernard's Hospital School of Nursing, Chicago,
Illinois, June 1947
BS Nursing Education, Loyola University, Chicago, Illinois,
June 1947 (concurrent with receipt of diploma from St.
Bernard's)
MS Nursing Education, Catholic University, psychiatric nurs-
ing major, June 1952
MA Philosophy, Georgetown University, 1960
PhD Philosophy, Georgetown University, 1968

1

Historical Development of the Model

Paterson and Zderad began theorizing about the nature of nursing amidst the clamor within the profession to develop a scientific basis of nursing practice. During the 1950s and 1960s, many nurses began to ask fundamental questions regarding the nature of nursing. Many psychiatric nurses explored in particular the nature of the nurse-patient relationship and viewed nurse-patient relations as the central phenomenon to be addressed in nursing theory development. Newman (1983) suggests that the 1950s and 1960s were dominated by this focus in nursing theory development. This is certainly true of Paterson and Zderad's (1988) model.

It was during this time that Paterson and Zderad began their "dialogue with reality" (Zderad, 1978, p. 39), which they later called theorizing. They did not set out deliberately and consciously with the intention to develop nursing theory. Nonetheless, they both describe a certain unrest in their teaching that stemmed from including bits and pieces from many nonnursing disciplines as opposed to teaching from nursing's theoretical base. This spurred their efforts to develop the theoretical basis of nursing. They describe their process of theorizing as a slow evolution toward nursing theory. Paterson (1978) has described the process of theory development in nursing as "tortuous" (p. 49), by which she conveys the nonlinear and somewhat mazelike nature of humanistic nursing practice theory development. Theorizing is thus filled

3

with meanderings, scenic paths, and seeming detours. Yet it remains intent upon seeking a clearing in the maze, an articulated vision of the reality of the lived nursing act.

Early in theory development, Paterson and Zderad became disillusioned with what they felt was an overemphasis on scientific processes of theory building. They did not feel that this scientific theory-building process was able to express fully the complexity or the aesthetic qualities of the nursing situation. Paterson and Zderad therefore developed a process of theorizing that was more akin to the nature of nursing itself.

> By analogy the model or form or phases of this method can be correlated with the model or form or phases of a clinical nursing process. This is an attempt to apply a method of study to nursing which corresponds to the nature of nursing as perceived by this author . . . this is a subjective-objective method of study that conforms to the nature of professional nursing. It attempts to describe the nature of the complex mobile spirit of nursing by a process which preserves this spirit intact. (Paterson, 1971, pp. 143, 146)

Therefore they experienced what all theorists, writers, and artists experience to some degree: namely, the limitations of words or images to convey the fullness of human experience. A quote by Bergson conveys their concern with this: "Fixed concepts can be extracted from our thought from the mobile reality; but there is no means whatever of reconstituting with the fixity of concepts the mobility of the real" (Bergson, 1962, cited in Paterson, 1971, p. 144). This concern led them to examine the discipline of philosophy wherein they learned different ways to explore the nature of things. They soon recognized their concerns as being more consistent with a phenomenological method of inquiry as compared with the scientific method. Later, they formulated a position that viewed phenomenological inquiry and scientific inquiry as complementary (Paterson & Zderad, 1978). Both theorists began the process of theorizing about nursing while actively engaged in the practices of clinical nursing and nursing education. The need to "root" (Zderad, 1978, p. 35) nursing theory in the clinical setting was another major goal of the theorists. Paterson (1978) describes theory and practice as "two sides of one indivisible coin" (p. 51). The threefold process of (a) experiencing, (b) reflecting upon, and (c) describing their nursing experiences emerged from their conscious attentiveness to the nature and meaning of these practices and ultimately became the cornerstone of the process of clinical theorizing that they termed *nursology* (Paterson, 1971). Recognition of and cultivation of the interrelationships of nursing practice, nursing education, and nursing research became both a hallmark of and the goal of humanistic nursing practice theory development. Indeed, the culmination of their careers as "nursologists" at the Northport Veterans Administration Hospital enabled them to engage simultaneously (all at once) in the three-pronged practices of clinical nursing (practice, education, and research) as they lived and articulated their vision of humanistic nursing practice theory.

Thus the theorizing efforts of Paterson and Zderad began with the recognition at some level that they themselves are, and indeed each practicing nurse is, a "noetic locus" (Desan, 1972, cited in Paterson & Zderad, 1988, p. 39), or a knowing place. It is the professional responsibility of each nurse to contribute to the evolution of nursing theory by attending knowingly to his or her practice and by asking questions of that practice—such as what, why, how, how better, ought, and ought not—by reflecting on possibilities and by articulating this vision in an enduring form to be shared both with other nurses and with humanity in general (Paterson & Zderad, 1978). Through such thoughtful attending and sharing by each nurse, a wide variety of nursing experiences can be brought under the umbrella of fewer enduring phenomena that will reflect the essential core of nursing as it is lived across diverse nursing contexts.

Staying with a chosen phenomenon over time by weaving back and forth between the experiencing, reflecting, and describing realms will generate rich phenomenological descriptions of essential nursing concepts and will reveal the relatedness among these concepts. The development of humanistic nursing practice theory proceeded along just these lines as Paterson and Zderad engaged themselves with in-depth study of their initially chosen and ever-evolving phenomena of interest. For example, Paterson began studying the phenomenon of ambivalence, moved through such concepts as growth, health, freedom, openness promotion, and, finally, focused on the concept of comfort (Paterson & Zderad, 1978). Zderad began with wondering how it is possible to know another person and traveled through such phenomena as empathy and presence to the notion of "withness" (Zderad, 1978, p. 44). The fruits of their individual and collective efforts are expressed as their major text, *Humanistic Nursing*, first published in 1976 and reprinted in 1988. The text is presented by the theorists as the culmination of their experience of teaching a continuing education course titled "Humanistic Nursing" at the Northport Veterans Administration Hospital over a period of years.

The development of humanistic nursing practice theory by Paterson and Zderad was thus a response to a call from within themselves to search for and to articulate the meaning and value of their own nursing practices. Nursing "undescribed and unappreciated" (Paterson, 1978, p. 51) is nursing inadequately conceptualized and uncommunicated to others. Thus their personal call resonated with the call within the profession of nursing to explicate the nature and significance of nursing as a professional discipline. Paterson and Zderad were thus among the pioneers in nursing who readily understood the value and nature of theory in a practice discipline and responded by developing a method of theorizing that is congruent with the practice of nursing.

The capstone summary statement of their view of theory is that of R. D. Laing, who stated that "theory is the articulated vision of experience" (Zderad, 1978, p. 45). Zderad stresses the meaning of each key word in Laing's definition. She states that *articulated* means that the theory is expressed in an enduring form so that it can be shared with others and also means that the connectedness among the concepts in the theory is evident. *Vision* refers to the heuristic nature of the theory; it calls us forth to enact the possibilities as envisioned by the theory and goes beyond merely summarizing past concrete experiences. *Experience* refers to the nurse's lived acts as a nurse in the health-illness community from multiple vantage points. Finally, they maintain that nursing theory is a valued resource for nurses as educators, practitioners, and researchers and for humanity in general.

In their seminal work, *Humanistic Nursing*, Paterson and Zderad convey their vision of nursing expressed as humanistic nursing practice theory and as a general theory of nursing. In addition, they provide a rich metatheoretical landscape from which other theories can be sculpted. Paterson (1978) defined *metatheory* as a "systematized body of knowledge formulated for the purpose of making something else possible" (p. 50). The most general forms of nursing's phenomena of concern have been asserted by some nursing scholars

(Fawcett, 1980, 1984; Flaskerud & Halloran, 1980; Newman, 1983) to form the metaparadigm of nursing. Flaskerud and Halloran (1980) have termed the four elements of nurse, person, health, and environment areas of agreement in nursing theory; that is, across time, these elements have formed the substance of nursing theory. It is common in nursing theory discourse to refer to metatheory as a conceptual framework. According to Fawcett (1980, 1984), a conceptual framework of nursing provides a distinct perspective on the elements of nursing's metaparadigm: namely, person, nursing, health, and environment. The perspective of Paterson and Zderad on the elements of the metaparadigm will now be presented. This presentation will be followed by a discussion of their general theory of nursing. This division is consistent with the theorists' assertion that there are two levels of nursing theorizing. The first is the phase of conceptualizing significant nursing phenomena phenomenologically. The second is the phase of interrelating the concepts into a coherent whole (Zderad, 1978, p. 45). The metatheory is more highly developed by the theorists than is the general theory of nursing. Nonetheless, the major concepts that are identified and explored within the metatheory are readily identified within the general theory of nursing.

Overview of Metatheory

Humanistic nursing as a metatheory of nursing provides highly developed viewpoints on the two metaparadigm elements of nursing and person and less well-developed views of health and environment. The development of the view of nursing as a particular kind of human relating is perhaps its major contribution. The essence of the metatheory provides "a perspective of nursing as a happening between persons, an approach to nursing as existential presence and awareness, and a method of describing nursing as phenomenology" (Paterson, 1978, p. 49). This statement provides insight on the assumptions that are implicit within the metatheory. *Assumptions* are assertions of basic beliefs that "are taken as givens" (Fawcett, 1984, p. 2) prior to the presentation of the major ideas within the metatheory. Assumptions reflect philosophical positions about human ways of being, knowing, and doing. Within the metatheory, several implicit assumptions can be discerned;

none has been deliberately put forward by the theorists as assumptions. They do, however, make the following comments regarding an apt starting point for humanistic nursing practice theory:

> Nursing situations make available human existence events significantly worthy of description. Only human nurses can describe them. Humans' ability to describe reality adequately has its limits. We should describe since pridefully we humans are the only existing beings capable of giving meaning to, looking at, and expressing our consciousness. In the long run this effort could yield a nursing science. (Paterson & Zderad, 1988, p. 70)

2

Implicit Assumptions

Nature of Reality

For Paterson and Zderad (1978), the nature of nursing reality is held to be objective, subjective, and intersubjective all at once. Objective reality can be thought of as occurring "out there" (Paterson & Zderad, 1978). It can be observed, pointed at, held at a distance, and examined. An object can be "apprehended intellectually" (Paterson & Zderad, 1988, p. 27). Subjective reality is known from the inside out; it is the reality that can be thought of as awareness of one's own experience. Intersubjective reality is experienced in what Paterson and Zderad term the *between* (Paterson & Zderad, 1988, p. 4). Intersubjective reality can be thought of as subject-to-subject relating. One's inherent capacity to respond to other beings-as-beings is what gives rise to the realm of the between as a facet of reality.

Humanistic nursing dwells primarily in the intersubjective realm of nursing even while recognizing the trifold (objective, subjective, intersubjective) nature of the nursing world. Similarly, the meta-theory seems to accentuate the "being" qualities of nursing even while recognizing the integrality of its "being and doing" (Paterson & Zderad, 1988, p. 13). At the time that they were developing their theory, Paterson and Zderad felt that the "doing" aspects of nursing had been more commonly examined.

9

It is not difficult to follow the evolution of Zderad's journey from empathy through presence toward "withness" as a central phenomenon of inquiry; the preposition *with* thus becomes central within the metatheory. *With* also becomes a central concept within the intersubjective realm. Nonetheless, it is important to underscore that these aspects of nursing that come under closer scrutiny within the metatheory are not held to exhaust the reality of the nursing world as it is lived. Objective reality and doing with patients continue to be viewed as appropriate ways of knowing and being in the nursing world.

One Becomes Ever More

Another basic belief that underpins the metatheory is that the nature of person is both to be and to become ever more. The "beingness" of persons will be discussed within the metatheory under "adequacy." Adequacy is one aspect of their view of the person. This basic belief also gives rise to two other related concepts within the metatheory known as "well-being" and "more-being," which speak to persons being and becoming ever more, respectively. These are discussed as health-related terms within the metatheory.

These and other basic beliefs within the metatheory can best be understood by examining the philosophical tenets of existentialism and phenomenology. Thinkers holding these philosophical views clearly influenced the development of Paterson and Zderad's thinking as did the two psychiatric mental health nurses Theresa G. Muller and Ruth Gilbert (Paterson & Zderad, 1988, p. 96). Nonetheless, the theorists' basic position on knowing underscores the new synthesis of thought that occurs within the knower through repeated cycles of experiencing, reflecting, and describing. The knower as a "noetic locus" synthesizes the thoughts of others with his or her own experience and reflection, giving rise to a new creation. Thus humanistic nursing practice theory should not be construed as an application of existential thought and phenomenological method within nursing as much as the "complementary synthesis" (1988, p. 73).

Humanistic nursing practice theory can be thought of as a blossoming of existential-phenomenological thought rather than as the plant that is firmly rooted in such thought. Nonetheless, as Paterson and Zderad (1978) maintain, while one can move from a philosophy to a theory realm, one cannot take the philosophy out of humanistic nursing practice theory. Persons are their history (past) as well as their choices (future); thus the theory is both distinct from and also related to the line of thought from which it arose.

The name given to this process of theorizing and to the resultant body of abstract knowledge in which it will ultimately result is *nursology*. The title given to nurses who undertake its development is *nursologist*.

Summary of Existential Thought

One thinker who is commonly associated with existentialism and who consents to be grouped with existentialists is Jean-Paul Sartre (1948, cited in White, 1983). According to Sartre (1948, cited in White, 1983), the central theme of existentialism is that *"existence* comes before *essence"* (p. 122). Existentialists believe that human beings do not have any predetermined nature or ultimate essence that thinkers through the years have called "human nature." Individuals are thus neither ultimately good nor ultimately evil. Instead, they come into the world and become all they will be based on choices that they continually make. They are not fulfilling any grand plan but are constantly free to make whatever choices they will. Paterson and Zderad (1988) depict the human as "lacking a fixed nature with his [or her] own mode of being as his [or her] fundamental project" (p. 78). This idea is commonly referred to as being "thrown" into the world and it underscores the freedom within the human condition. Sartre speaks of this "terrible freedom" (Sartre, cited in Guigan, 1986) that results from realization that individuals are free to become who they will. Coupled with this individual freedom is the responsibility for personal choices and this gives rise to the other central themes in existential thought: anxiety, dread, and abandonment. Capability unrealized is not treasured in this viewpoint. Sartre (1948, cited in White, 1983) states that, in the final analysis, "man [*sic*] is no other than a series of undertakings, that he [or she] is the sum, the organization, the set of relations that constitute these undertakings" (p. 135).

Many existential thinkers highlight the redemptive value of human relatedness. If it is one's plight to endure the "terrible freedom," it is also one's promise to do so in the company of others. Thus an important theme in existential writings is one's relation to others and one's responsibility to cultivate communities of dialogue. Dialogue becomes the primary way to experience community. The existential experience thus becomes one of both solitude and solidarity, which is perhaps the central paradox within existential thought.

Threads of existential thought can be seen in the centrality of choice within the metatheory of Paterson and Zderad (1988). They also espouse the primacy of action perspective that is essential to such thought. For example, they treasure the practices of humanistic nursing and highlight their interrelatedness to the knowing aspects of nursing. Finally, their general theory of nursing rests on a central premise of existential thought, that of the possibility of individual growth through authentic relating.

The use of the term *humanistic nursing* to describe their continuing education class was deliberately chosen by the theorists after first experimenting with longer titles that included the term *phenomenology*. The theorists (1988) state that they used the term *humanistic* to refer to an approach that encompasses an existential concept of person and a phenomenological approach to inquiry. Furthermore, they intended for this term to convey all ways of being and becoming. The place of technology is not negated in the use of the term *humanistic nursing*. Instead, technology is seen to be a human capability.

Summary of Phenomenological Tradition

The central slogan of the phenomenological tradition might be held to be "to the things themselves." This saying is attributed to Husserl, the father of phenomenology (Paterson & Zderad, 1988). Phenomenological methods are primarily concerned with describing human experience in such a way that the fullness of experience is preserved. These methods cultivate knowing from within an experience rather than from looking at the experience from the outside.

For Paterson and Zderad (1988), the lived nursing act thus becomes the "thing itself" to which nursing theory must return.

These lived acts of nursing become the fountainhead of humanistic nursing practice theory. The acts, when subjected to phenomenological description and inquiry by the community of nurses over time, will reveal the phenomena of central concern to nursing as a practice discipline. Paterson and Zderad's phenomenological method of nursology will be further described within their view of nursing as knowing.

3

---

*Perspectives on
Metaparadigm Elements*

Person

Paterson and Zderad's view of persons is meant to apply to both the nurse and the patient and can be thought of as fleshing out their implicit assumptions. Within the metatheory, the patient is commonly referred to as *the nursed*. The use of this term underscores aspects of persons with which nurses are distinctly concerned, namely, persons-as-nursed. The use of the term also underscores the relational quality of the nurse-nursed relationship. One of the most important features of their view of persons is that they distinguish between ways of being-as-nurse and being-as-patient. This has implications for their conceptualization of nursing as a distinct form of human relating that is both similar to and yet distinct from other forms of human relating.

Freedom

According to Paterson and Zderad (1988), a major aspect of human nature is its nondeterminedness. Closely related to this premise is the notion that humans are "responsible for their condition of being" (Paterson & Zderad, 1988, p. 3). As a person, "I am my choices"

(Paterson & Zderad, 1988, p. 15). Paterson and Zderad interpret this existential dictum to mean that persons have an inherent capacity to choose to respond and to choose how to respond to situations presented by life. Therefore a person is not seen as choosing the situation but is held accountable for personal response to it. While this response influences the emerging situation as it changes over time, the response alone is an insufficient determinant of the health or illness situation. This distinction is important when considering the health and illness quality of life, because health and illness are influenced by multiple other factors not within the realm of individual accountability such as heredity, exposure to environmental agents, or natural disasters. The description of choice within Paterson and Zderad's (1988) conceptual model occurs in three phases. Phase 1 of the choice process is an awareness phase in which one recognizes that possibilities exist. In other words, the possibilities must become relevant. This openness to possibility is characterized by a freedom from "the bonds of habit and stereotyped response" (Paterson & Zderad, 1988, p. 16) and conveys a sense of openness to spontaneity and availability. In addition, this first phase of choice involves "getting in touch with one's experience, one's subjective-objective world" (Paterson & Zderad, 1988, p. 16) and one's situation. In phase 2, one engages in reflection. In this phase of choice, one considers one's "unique situation . . . possible alternatives, . . . the values inherent within them" (Paterson & Zderad, 1988, p. 16). This reflection bears elements of the past (values), the current time (unique situation), and the future (possible alternatives). Finally, the person responds with a choice that is "expressed . . . as a willingness to accept responsibility for its foreseeable consequences" (Paterson & Zderad, 1988, p. 16).

Uniqueness

Paterson and Zderad underscore the distinctiveness of the person. Every person holds his or her own "angular view" (Paterson & Zderad, 1988, p. 37). This refers to the fact that every person sees, hears, feels, tastes, and experiences the world differently. These different experiences, which include the influence of family and history, give rise to a particular viewpoint or way of seeing the world.

Another belief of Paterson and Zderad (1988) regarding human nature is that, while every person is unique, it is this shared fact of uniqueness that persons have in common with each other. This uniqueness results in choices that appear somewhat lonely in that "only each person can describe or choose the evolvement of the project which is himself-in-his-situation" (Paterson & Zderad, 1988, p. 4).

Adequacy

While human choice might be lonely, it is also linked to the critical human capacity of hope, which inspires one to envision alternatives beyond those immediately apparent. While envisioning possibilities, one is confronted by conflicting and seemingly competing alternatives as well as by human limitation. Paterson and Zderad (1988) refer to the resolution of the polarity of human potential and limitation as "humanness," or the notion that it is "just how man [sic] is" (Paterson & Zderad, 1988, p. 5). *Humanness* also refers to the presence within humans of "the spiritual and the animal" (Paterson & Zderad, 1988, p. 55). Elsewhere, Paterson (1978) refers to this aspect of persons as a sense of human "adequacy" (p. 54).

Relatedness

Finally, one's capacity for relationship with others is a key attribute of individuals within this metatheory. This capacity for person-to-person relating Paterson and Zderad (1988) discuss as a capacity for presence, or being with another human being. Through relating with other persons as presences (intersubjectivity), individuals become more and realize their uniqueness. The choice to relate in such a way is made deliberately. Thus two interrelated processes are seen by Paterson and Zderad to contribute to human moreness, namely, choice and intersubjectivity.

Historicity

Nurses are their history and of necessity this affects their inner responses to their nursing world. Awareness of the meaning of their personal history enables them to be "in charge of it" (Paterson, 1978, p. 63) rather than for it to be in charge of them. Being in charge also applies to patients. Historicity contributes to the situatedness of choice. Thus one can choose within the limits of what one sees as possibilities. Part of the nursing process is engaging the patient's capacity to envision for him- or herself unseen possibilities.

Person-as-Nurse

Person-as-nurse is one who responds to the call of human beings with needs within the health-illness quality of life. According to Paterson (1978), nursing is a unique way of responding that will continue as a human response even if the nursing profession were to stop using the word *nursing* to describe its activity. Paterson (1978) also maintains that nursing as a profession survives because all humans have the potential to become patients.

Person-as-nurse is a presence with others whose health and survival are at issue. According to Paterson (1978), the nurse's existence is confirmed because of the difference made in the situation. Therefore person-as-nurse needs to nurse just as person-as-patient (nursed) needs to be nursed. Furthermore, a person-as-nurse identifies with the profession and is responsible to it. Person-as-nurse is therefore committed to strive to express the fullest meaning of humanistic nursing, which is seen as "existential engagement directed toward nurturing human potential" (Paterson & Zderad, 1988, p. 14). The key idea is that the nurse's commitment is to strive continually toward humanistic nursing as a goal despite the fact that in practice it may occur in various degrees.

Person-as-Patient

Within the metatheory, the person-as-patient is referred to as "the nursed" (Paterson & Zderad, 1978). The theorists assert that, because of the limitations inherent in the human condition, we all have the capacity to become patients. Paterson states,

> To be a patient is to worry, hurt, and suffer to a degree beyond one's own ability to heal or bear alone . . . I am a being in a body; through my body my being is touched and affected. Because of this body it is necessary to lean, to depend. I am very aware of and alert to those other beings who touch and affect me, who support me. . . . I may experience them as being more or less powerful or benevolent than they really are. (1978, pp. 54-55)

Nursing

paradigm element of nursing is the most highly devel-
opea ~ within the metatheory. Thus several different views of
nursing are found within the metatheory. Integral to the theorists'
thinking is that nursing is a way of knowing, being, and doing.

The most general view about nursing is that the three practice
realms in nursing (education, practice, and research) are intimately
connected and together constitute clinical nursing. Paterson and
Zderad (1988) maintain that humanistic nursing is concerned "with
the phenomenon of nursing wherever it occurs regardless of its
specialized clinical, functional or sociocultural form" (p. 18). Knowing and doing are thus interconnected processes that cut across all
aspects of clinical nursing. Nursology is the successful weaving
together of the three strands of clinical nursing.

Nursing as Knowing

Nursing as art-science. The notion of nursing as art-science is
meant to convey the interrelated processes of art and science as
they occur all at once in the nursing situation. Even the hyphen
does not convey the synthesis of art and science that Paterson and
Zderad hold as integral to nursing. They define the art-science
quality of nursing as "a symbolic behavioral expression of intuitive
logical knowledge derived from subjective, objective, and intersubjective experiences with reality" (1978). The notion of art-science highlights the multifaceted nature of knowing in nursing.

Nursing as a unique knowledge form. Highlighting the dynamic of
distinctiveness within relatedness, Paterson and Zderad take the
position that *nursing* used as a noun is a unique form of knowledge
yet is related to general knowledge. The unique contribution of
nursing to human science is expressed first in a question: "What
knowledge gained through the study of nursing, a particular form
of the human situation, could be contributed to the general body
of human sciences?" (Paterson & Zderad, 1976, p. 20). Later in the
metatheory, the unique knowledge of nursing and its potential
contribution to general knowledge are expressed in the uniqueness
of the dialogical process of nursing as it occurs through nursing

acts. The potential contribution of nursing to general knowledge of dialogical human processes is "staggering" (Paterson & Zderad, 1976, p. 34). It is a combination of being with and doing with the patient in the nursing situation.

The value of conceptualizing this knowledge, embodied within concrete practice situations, and of articulating it in enduring form is echoed repeatedly by the theorists. For example, Zderad (1978) states: "Nursing, as every discipline, has its own distinctive encounter with reality; and in its encounter, each seeks meaning" (p. 48). This meaning in nursing science reflects both a body of substantive knowledge and a method for discovering and verifying new knowledge. "Each science, then, bears these twin hallmarks: its particular area of concern with reality and its particular approach to theorizing about it" (Zderad, 1978, p. 48). These concrete practice descriptions are seen as building blocks for nursing science. Articulation of the unique knowledge of nursing, however, is seen by Paterson and Zderad to have yet broader ramifications for human knowledge development: "If we truly experience nursing as a kind of art-science, as a particular dyad of flowing, synthesizing, subjective-objective intersubjective dialogue, then nursing offers a unique path to human knowledge and it is our responsibility to try to describe and share it" (1976, p. 102).

Nursology. Nursology is the name given to a process of scientific inquiry in nursing that was first introduced by Paterson in 1971. She defined it as "the study of nursing aimed towards the development of nursing theory" (1971, p. 143). While viewed by Paterson as a form of phenomenology, it was also seen as a new creation that resulted from a "complementary synthesis" (p. 73) of phenomenological thought and nursing experience.

The method of nursology surfaced in true phenomenological fashion after Paterson reflected upon her experiences of trying to conceptualize the term *clinical.* Intent upon the outcome of her conceptualization of this term, the process by which this occurred went largely unnoticed. Of interest, it was the elucidation of the process of conceptualizing known as *nursology* that made its more enduring impact on nursing than the original conceptualization of the term *clinical.* The process of inquiry known as *nursology* is among the forerunners of methodologies distinct to nursing science. Paterson and Zderad were pioneers among nurse scholars in recognizing the need for congruence in philosophy, science, and method. The tradition has continued in nursing science with Parse's (1987) Man-Living-Health research methodology, a variant of phenomenology, and Leininger's (1985) ethnonursing method, which is derived from ethnographic methods.

A noteworthy characteristic of nursology is its similarity to the practice of clinical nursing. This view is consistent with Paterson and Zderad's beliefs in the integrality of nursing education, research, and clinical practice. Thus research was not held as something to be conducted only by academics but as part of the lived experience of all professional nurses, who weave the three threads of knowing, being, and doing into the art-science of practice.

The method of nursology seeks to answer the following question: "How can the nurse, a subjective-objective human being, know the other, be it person, thing, or spirit, and compare and complementarily synthesize these known others?" (Paterson, 1971, p. 144). The five overlapping and nonsequential phases of the method are (a) preparation of the knower for knowing, (b) knowing the other intuitively, (c) knowing the other scientifically, (d) complementarily synthesizing known others, and (e) succeeding from the "many" to the "paradoxical one" (Paterson, 1971, pp. 144-145; Paterson & Zderad, 1988, pp. 70-74).

Phase 1 (preparation of the knower) is a phase of receptivity and openness on the part of the knower. It is not a passive waiting but an active response to the invitation to know. The knower embraces an attitude of inquisitiveness and hopefulness and resists habitual response within situations. Paterson (1971) describes this as a risk-taking phase in which one dares to see the world as it presents itself rather than through an already established theoretical scheme. The "bracketing" (holding in abeyance) of one's prior assumptions, categories, and conceptions is attempted in this phase, although the impossibility of attaining a state of being without perspective is readily acknowledged. Instead, one attempts to gain maximal awareness of one's "angular view" such that one's shaded view of reality is recognized and considered. The outcome of this phase is the recognition and presentation of one's angular view of something.

Phase 2 (knowing the other intuitively) refers to the intuitive aspects of knowing in which the knower grasps the whole of the other through an imaginative process of getting in touch with the other's "rhythm and mobility" (Paterson, 1971, p. 144). The knower does not analyze the other. Intuition comes in the form of insight and understanding while analysis comes through a deliberate process of explaining or examining the other. This phase of knowing is comparable to the "I-Thou" moment in the transactive nursing process. Citing Buber, Paterson (1971, p. 144) states that intuitive-type knowing requires an "I" capable of both distance and relation with the other. The combination of distance and relation highlights the tension between merging with the other and maintaining a sense of one's own distinctiveness from the other. In this phase of knowing, the knower "does not superimpose, maintains a capacity for surprise and question, and is with the other as opposed to 'seeming to be' " (Paterson, 1971, p. 144). This intuitive phase necessarily precedes any meaningful analytic phase.

Phase 3 (knowing the other scientifically) highlights the kind of knowing that is a "looking at." It compares with the "I-It" moments in the transactive nursing process wherein the other is held at a distance and examined in its objectness. It is a phase of analysis and of interpretation. In this phase, a "name" is given to the lived experience and it is seen no longer primarily in its uniqueness but in its similarities to and differences from other experiences. It may become part of a categorization scheme. Its outcome is a relatively fixed symbolic representation of what had been the "mobile reality" (Bergson, cited in Paterson, 1971, p. 144) of the nursing situation.

Phase 4 (complementary synthesis) is the phase in which the knower as "noetic locus" (Paterson, 1971, p. 145) conducts an internal dialogue between the singular reality as conceptualized in Phase 3 and multiple other known realities. Within the knower, similarities and differences are noted among the multiple realities and a new creation emerges from this internal dialogue. This dialogue may lead to a statement of a general principle that includes, but is not exhausted by, the original experience. Complementary synthesis is thus described as "being more than additive because it allows mutual representation and illumination of one reality by another" (Paterson & Zderad, 1988, p. 74). In nursing process, this phase is likened to the noting of similarities and differences by the nurse across individual patients or within individual patients over time.

The fifth and final phase of nursology—succession from the "We" (Paterson, 1971, p. 145) or the "many" (Paterson & Zderad, 1988, p. 74) to the "paradoxical one"—refers to the phase in which the knower's original angular view of the other is changed as a result of participation in the first four phases of knowing. It is an acknowledgment of the transformative power of knowing. Its form is to be "ever more inclusive" (Paterson & Zderad, 1988, p. 74). This statement means that the transformed view of the other includes, but is not exhausted by, the newly formed insight. It is a view from the other side of the paradox that is obtained by struggling through the multiplicities toward a unified insight that moves knowledge forward. This temporary resting place can be likened to a moment of well-being in knowing; a moment in which the struggle to move beyond the achieved insight is suspended until one confronts in the clinical world something that cannot be included within the insight. Then begins the struggle toward more-being in knowing as the continuous refrain begins yet again.

Nursing as Doing and Being

Nursing as presence. Paterson and Zderad (1988) were among the first nursing theorists to explicate the concept of presence in nursing. Zderad (1978) suggests that the phenomenon as experienced in nursing situations is distinct from, yet related to, the phenomenon in general.

> Its occurrence or absence can be experienced. Both nurse and patient are aware of it. It is important to both. It makes one aware of oneself and of the other. It reveals a person to himself and to the other. Through it the nurse and the patient can show respect, closeness, caring—in short can confirm each other. In nurse-patient situations, the nurse's presence is expected by both. . . . [I]s "presence" a depreciable intangible in nursing that is more obvious in its absence? (Zderad, 1978, p. 42)

The theorists maintain that presence in nursing is a most exquisite rendition of "being with and doing with" (Paterson & Zderad, 1976, p. 13) patients. They suggest that "doing" aspects had previously been described in nursing. Their discussion of presence therefore focused on the quality of the nurse's being while recognizing that one of the distinct features of being present as a nurse is the inextricability of the threads of both being and doing. They further clarify the nature of this quality of being (which is expressed also in the doing) as involving one's whole being, as being given freely and chosen freely, and as being both personal and professional. The personal dimension attests to the unique quality of presence that each nurse brings to the nursing situation given her "angular" (Paterson & Zderad, 1976, p. 37) or unique perspective. Professional quality refers both to the goal-directedness of the situation and to the professional accountability of the nurse. Paterson and Zderad see nursing as being goal directed. The goal is "nurturing well-being and more-being" (Paterson & Zderad, 1976, p. 28) of patients within the "domain of health and illness" (p. 28). The accountability of the nurse to the patient, while experienced personally as human to human, is magnified and colored by the professional nature of the relationship. This professional accountability is influenced by the "limits of safe and sound practice" (Paterson & Zderad, 1976, p. 17) and is manifested by the nurse's "responsible choosing of overt responses based in knowledge and on nursing values" (Paterson & Zderad, 1976, p. 57).

A particularly important contribution of Paterson and Zderad's discussion of presence in the nursing situation is its ability to limit the concept within nursing's scope. The boundedness of the concept of presence is perhaps best seen in Paterson and Zderad's (1988) discussion of the attributes of presence such as spontaneity, availability, reciprocity, and mutuality. While the foregoing are seen as critical attributes of presence, they are distinctly colored by the purpose of the nursing situation.

Paterson and Zderad's discussion of the attribute of spontaneity suggests their recognition of the tension between the goal-directedness of professional nursing presence and the inability to call forth presence on demand. Instead, presence can only be invoked or evoked and is a "gift of oneself" (Paterson & Zderad, 1988, p. 16) that is "revealed in a glance, touch or tone of voice" (Paterson & Zderad, 1988, p. 88). Therefore, immediately preceding presence, they recognize a "certain openness, a receptivity, readiness or availability" (Paterson & Zderad, 1988, p. 28). Said another way, being with in its fullest sense (presence) requires "turning one's attention toward the patient, being aware of and open to the here and now shared situation and communicating one's availability" (Paterson & Zderad, 1988, p. 14). It is the goal-directed nature of the nursing situation that modifies the quality of the availability, spontaneity, reciprocity, and mutuality that characterize nursing presence. *Availability* is modified as "availability-in-a-helping-way"

(Paterson & Zderad, 1976, p. 28) and *openness* becomes an "openness to a person-with-needs" (Paterson & Zderad, 1976, p. 28).

Reciprocity, another critical attribute of nursing presence, is described as seeing both nurse (self) and patient (other) "as persons rather than as objects or functions" (Paterson & Zderad, 1988, p. 28). This reciprocity does not require that no differences be recognized between the presence of the nurse and the presence of the patient. Rather, the professional quality of nursing presence is "somehow colored by a sense of responsibility or regard for what is seen as the patient's vulnerability" (Paterson & Zderad, 1988, p. 28). The mutuality that characterizes nursing presence is not so much one of equality or of being "shared alike" as would be suggested by dictionary definitions of the term. Rather, reciprocity is seen as "flow between two persons with different modes of being in the shared situation" (Paterson & Zderad, 1988, p. 29).

Nursing as dialogue. The notion of nursing as dialogue conveys the back and forth ebb and flow of nursing as conveyed by Paterson and Zderad. Nursing cannot take place without the nursed. Within this image of nursing, the theorists discuss nursing lived as a "purposeful call and response" (Paterson & Zderad, 1988, p. 29). They state:

> Nursing implies a special kind of meeting of human persons. It occurs in response to a perceived need related to the health-illness quality of the human condition. Within that domain, . . . nursing is directed toward the goal of nurturing well-being and more-being (human potential). Nursing, therefore, does not involve a merely fortuitous encounter, but rather one in which there is purposeful call and response. In this vein, humanistic nursing may be considered a special kind of lived dialogue. (1988, p. 24)

This discussion again calls attention to the fact that, for Paterson and Zderad, the mutuality that is involved in the nursing situation is experienced differently by the nurse and the nursed. This belief underscores the different modes of being in the situation that both bring.

They further describe dialogical nursing as a "transactive" process. By this description, they mean to convey the fact that the nursing process goes "both ways" (Paterson & Zderad, 1976, p. 132) between the participants (the nurse and the nursed). Even in

the "intervention" phase of nursing, the nurse can
possibilities seen within the patient, but "the patient
ipate as an active subject to actualize the possibility (fc
himself [or herself]" (Paterson & Zderad, 1988, p. 92). Th _ünin
the transaction, there is always call and response. In another example, the theorists highlight the mutuality of the relation. They
state, "Not only does the nurse see the possibilities in the patient
but the patient also sees a form in the nurse (for example, possibility of help, of comfort, of support), and he [or she] responds in
relation to bring it forth" (Paterson & Zderad, 1988, p. 92). In
addition, they point out that the meaning of acts that occur in
nursing situations are different for the nurse and the nursed. For
instance, touch can be experienced as touching or being touched;
the experience of feeding as feeding or being fed.

Health

Paterson and Zderad raise fundamental questions about whether
health is the appropriate goal of nursing. They state that "the
nursing act is always related to the health-illness quality of the
human condition, or fundamentally to man's [*sic*] personal survival . . . that nursing is related to health and illness is self-evident.
How it is related is not so apparent" (1988, p. 12). Therefore they
acknowledge the obviousness of nursing's involvement in health
and illness but note that some of the most exquisite nursing acts
occur in situations whereby health, taken in its narrow sense as the
absence of disease, is not feasible as an aim. Some examples include dying patients, patients with incurable diseases, and those
with chronic health conditions.

Comfort

Other nurses who have noted the poor fit between the definition
of health as the absence of disease and nursing's focus have rede-
fined health to include other meanings. Smith (1981) has pointed
out some of these alternate meanings of health that have been
commonly used in nursing discourse. Paterson and Zderad, however, chose to define the aim of nursing as "comfort," which
became "an umbrella term under which all other [health-related]

terms could be sheltered" (1988, p. 99). They reasoned that *comfort* was a term of historical importance in nursing and stated that it was also discussed in an ANA publication of their era as being of particular importance. Furthermore, it was a term that suggested itself to them as they sought to understand the major value that underlined their nursing practices (Paterson & Zderad, 1988, p. 98). Comfort was not chosen at whim; it emerged as an answer to the question as to "why" nurses are present in the health-illness situation.

The notion of comfort conveyed the sense that persons can be comfortable without being healthy and it is the promotion of this comfortable way of being that reflects nursing's most immediate concern. In other words, no matter what the state of health of a patient, a state of more or less comfort exists that is the proper aim of nursing. A patient can "be with" his or her health situation in a more or less comfortable way; this perhaps anticipated the ANA's definition of nursing as being most concerned with the person's *response* to the health-illness situation (ANA, 1980).

The notion of comfort was also used to underscore the basic orientational belief that persons are capable of becoming ever more. The theorists state, "Nursing's concern is not only with the well-being but with the more-being of patients" (Paterson & Zderad, 1988, p. 12). Thus comfort conveys the notion that a human being is "all he [or she] could be in accordance with his [or her] potential at any particular time in any particular situation" (1988, p. 101).

Through their discussion of the similarities of the term *comfort* with the notion of contentment, Paterson and Zderad (1988) bring to light their particular understanding of the term *comfort*: It "does not imply passivity, resignation, retirement, or a simple avoiding of trouble" (Paterson & Zderad, 1988 p. 101). It is important that comfort not be equated with the absence of pain. While the absence of pain can certainly be a comfortable state, it does not exhaust its possibilities. Because of the human capacity to become ever more, the natural state of human comfort is one of striving. Nonetheless, because of the notion of human adequacy and the tension between adequacy and possibility, it does not become what Benner and Wrubel (1989) have called "effortful striving." Boredom or lack of challenge can be as uncomfortable to humans as physical pain. Paterson and Zderad readily acknowledge that nurses at times encourage patients to experience stress or anxiety in the interest of growth. Zbilut (1980) has pointed out that this approach is common in holistic nursing practice. Achieving comfort is not akin to taking the easy way out of a situation or avoidance, although these possibilities remain open.

The ethics of this existentially grounded approach to comfort promotion have been questioned by Stevens (1990). She worries about the nurse imposing an existential view of comfort on patients. Does adopting this view of comfort mean that every patient should confront his or her situation and struggle to find its meaning? What about therapeutic denial? The key is to remember that, while the nurse might invite the patient to consider different possibilities, the nurse does not impose them on the patient. The mutuality of the nursing process as portrayed by these theorists would not allow such imposition of the nurses' intention on the patient. Nor would the patient's state of comfort-discomfort be solely determined by the nurse as a nursing diagnosis. Instead, the comfort-discomfort experience of the patient might be discerned by the nurse and then must be validated by the patient. It is highly likely that comfort goals will vary greatly both between patients and within a given patient over time. The important thing is to remain open to variation and choice within different contexts and understandings of comfort rather than stipulating what comfort will be. How much choice and variation is enough or too much within a professional relationship remains an ethical question of extreme importance within the discipline of nursing and one that is not limited to the problems posed by the existential viewpoint. Paterson and Zderad's view of the nurse-nursed relation identifies some limits within which such freedom is exercised, both on the part of the nurse and on the part of the patient. This view is consistent with their basic belief in situated versus radical freedom.

Well-Being and More-Being

Well-being and *more-being* are related terms within the metatheory and refer to human actuality and potential. Both are seen to contribute to the overall level of comfort of a given patient. In fact, they represent the essential tension between being and becoming, between what is and what might be, that characterizes the person within this metatheory. Well-being is closely related to the understanding of persons as "adequate" as described above. There is a sense in which humans are enough or just so. In addition, humans are free to choose to become more. Moreness is therefore a chosen way of being. It cannot be superimposed from the outside. The chief way in which persons become more is through relating to other persons in the various ways of "I-Thou," "I-It," and "We" (Paterson & Zderad, 1988, p. 44).

Environment

Views of the environment are not as fully explicated within this conceptual model as are the views of person and nursing. Nonetheless, references to relationships with the world in unique situations can easily be discerned. Paterson and Zderad state: "Nursing takes place in the real world of men [sic] and things in time and space" (1988, p. 33). Further, they maintain that the meanings of these "things" vary between persons and that the time and space to which they refer are "as they are experienced" (Paterson & Zderad, 1988, p. 34). Human beings and the world are viewed as both distinct from each other and intimately related. Objective reality (something out there apart from one's experience of it) does exist even as subjective reality also exists. Paterson and Zderad (1988) thus avoid the idealist extreme of positing a *purely* subjective reality.

Despite the inclusion of objective reality, the main focus of Paterson and Zderad's view of the environment is that of time and space as experienced by both the patient and the nurse. Of particular concern is the subjective experience of both the patient and the nurse in a given situation such as crutch-walking or dealing with chronic illness and also with their intersubjective or shared experiences of the given situation (1988, p. 19). In addition, while they acknowledge the environmental aspects of the nursing situation, Paterson and Zderad continue to hold the intersubjective nursing relationship as being of primary concern.

Here-and-Now

Paterson and Zderad's concept of the here-and-now always concerns a respect for the connectedness among one's past, current time, and future. It is always inclusive of both the nurses' and the patients' "origin, history, hopes, fears, and alternatives" (1988, p. 68). Both participants in the nursing dialogue bring to the here-and-now their unique backgrounds and their hopes for the future. The notion of here-and-now builds upon the basic assumption of one's essential uniqueness and the responsibility this conveys. It can also refer to the fact that each here-and-now moment is significant and irreplaceable. Paterson and Zderad paraphrase Herman Hesse on this point, "Every nurse is more than just herself [or himself], she [or he] also represents the unique, the very special and always significant and remarkable point at which the nursing world's phenomena intersect, only once in this way and never again" (1988, p. 69). Therefore it is the responsibility of each nurse to contribute to the development of general knowledge and nursing science by contributing his or her "nursing here-and-now to nursing's history through a lasting form of expression" (Paterson & Zderad, 1988, p. 69).

Nursing Situation

The nursing situation is a backdrop against which the intersubjective transaction that characterizes nursing dialogue occurs. It is a backdrop that at times becomes woven into the intersubjective transaction. Thus, while the theorists "place at the center of [their] universe . . . the nurse-patient intersubjective transaction" (Paterson & Zderad, 1988, p. 36), they readily acknowledge that this relationship does not take place in a vacuum. Indeed, they state that the "nursing dialogue is subjected to all the chaotic forces of life" (1988, p. 31). Furthermore, they underscore that the health world is among the most complex, chaotic, and conflicted realms of existence. They present a summary statement of the nursing situation and hold it out as an inclusive yet open framework from which to explore more deeply the essential elements of humanistic nursing. They state that its elements would include "incarnate men [*sic*] (patient and nurse) meeting (being and becoming) in a goal-directed (nurturing well-being and more-being) intersubjective transaction (being with and doing with) occurring in time and space (measured and as lived by patient and nurse) in a world of men [*sic*] and things" (Paterson & Zderad, 1988, p. 18). Thus they readily afford to the environment a subjective and intersubjective nature ("as lived") and also an objective quality ("world of men and things") that must be reckoned with.

Included within the nursing situation is the effect of other human beings on both the nurse and the nursed. The participants' network of significant others influences the immediate nurse-patient situation. They state that the current lived nursing dialogue is "always colored by the patient's current mode of interpersonal relating" (Paterson & Zderad, 1988, p. 32). This statement further supports the inclusion of past and future elements in the here-and-now.

"Things" are also a significant part of the nursing situation within the metatheory. Not only does nursing dialogue take place in a "real world of men [sic] and things" (Paterson & Zderad, 1988, p. 32), but these ordinary things often take on a different significance in the nursing situation because of their connection to the health-illness quality of life and because of the different ways of being in the situation as nurse and patient. For example, because of a health-illness situation, the patient may at times attribute great significance to ordinary things previously taken for granted, such as being able to use a knife or fork. Likewise, the nurse's familiar things include machines and instruments and use of space in ways that are not familiar to patients. Both the individual and the shared meanings of the things that are in the situation are highly significant within humanistic nursing. For example, the humanistic nurse might take special precaution to avoid "medicalizing" familiar things within the patient's world such as food and drink. Judicious use of both medical and lay terminology is needed in humanistic nursing practice.

All-at-Once

All-at-once is a pivotal concept within the metatheory. It is the primary way in which the theorists convey both the paradoxical nature of human reality and the complex reality of the nursing world. The many paradoxical qualities of humans include the fact that, while all persons are unique, they are also similar. Another important paradox is that the individual's capacities include virtue and vice, spiritual and animal qualities, that are experienced all-at-once. Paterson and Zderad state that "human existence in the world calls for an enduring with our virtues and vices, our energy and our laziness, our altruism and our selfishness, in a word with our humanness" (1988, p. 55). To deny either polarity as possibilities within ourselves or others results in a milieu of blame instead of one of responsibility and fosters a sense of powerlessness instead of well-being.

The use of the term *all-at-once* to communicate the complexity of the nursing situation is also common. This use underscores human existence as "never completely fathomable" (Paterson & Zderad, 1988, p. 8) and difficult to convey in words by use of strictly scientific processes of inquiry. As for the nursing situation, Paterson and Zderad use the term *multifarious multiplicities* to convey the complex web of occurrences that take place on a daily basis in everyday nursing situations. Nursing situations are "loaded with all kinds of incomparable data" (Paterson & Zderad, 1988, p. 96). Thus *all-at-once*, more than any other term, describes the "what" of the nursing situation and is used to describe its complexity. In fact, according to Paterson and Zderad, a hallmark of nursing skill is the ability to balance these multifarious multiplicities as they occur in the health world.

Finally, with regard to nurses' relating, the theorists use the notion of all-at-once to refer to the dual nature of nursing's engagement in the worlds of "I-Thou" and "I-It." They state that "the 'all-at-once' is equated by [us] to Buber's 'I-Thou' and 'I-It' occurring simultaneously and not only in sequence as he expressed it. These two ways that man [*sic*] can relate to and come to know his [or her] world and himself [or herself] demand sequential expression. . . . However, the responsible authentic nurse in the nursing arena lives them 'all-at-once' " (Paterson & Zderad, 1988, p. 110). The nursing world thus mirrors the essential tension between these two modes of relating and reflects a resolution of the tension in the all-at-once experience that is the lived nursing act.

Community

The nurse-patient relationship can be defined as a form of community given Paterson and Zderad's definition of *community* as "two or more persons struggling toward a common center" (1988, p. 121). Nonetheless, community is also portrayed as an element within which this relation unfolds.

When it is experienced as a "between" phenomenon, it is more readily experienced than explained. Paterson and Zderad's view of community values differences and does not seek conformity. In the experience of community, "discovered differences in similar realities do not compete, one does not negate the other. . . . Differences can make visible the greater realities of each" (Paterson & Zderad, 1988, p. 73).

Complementary Synthesis

This notion is highly related to the term *all-at-once*. It again refers to the fact that nursing's reality is a multiple one in which the nurse must traverse both the objective scientific world and the subjective and intersubjective realms of nursing situations. The tension between these realms is lived out in the nursing act. They state, "Doing with and being with the patient calls for a complementary synthesis by the nurse of these two forms of human dialogue, 'I-It' and 'I-Thou.' Both are inherent in humanistic nursing, for it is a dialogue lived in the objective and intersubjective realms of the real world" (Paterson & Zderad, 1988, p. 36).

In addition, this concept is also seen in Paterson and Zderad's process of inquiry. Complementary syntheses occur in both phases 4 and 5 of nursology. When used as part of the inquiry process, it refers to a process of attending to realities other than one's own "angular view." It thus is a form of communicating and connecting self and others and self and world. Thus the process of complementary synthesis characterizes both nursing situations and the process of nursology.

4

General Theory of Nursing

The second phase of theorizing, that of relating the explicated concepts, is illustrated by Paterson and Zderad's (1988) "theory of nursing" (p. 111). They propose relationships among their phenomenologically derived concepts. They state, "A human nurse nurses through a clinical process of I-Thou I-It all-at-once to comfort" (1988, p. 111). Though the concepts arose from psychiatric mental health nursing, the theorists assert that they are applicable across all nursing contexts. This affirmation illustrates a movement from the "many to the paradoxical one" (Paterson & Zderad, 1988, p. 74) whereby their particular conception of nursing is held to be meaningful to "the many or to all" (Paterson & Zderad, 1988, p. 75).

The specific form of the nursing relationship proposed by Paterson and Zderad is that of the "I-Thou, I-It, all-at once" (1988, p. 111). This relation can be described as a reformulation of Buber's (1953) "I-Thou" relationship. The reformulation is necessary to portray the unique aspects of relating within nursing situations. Specifically, the need to include some objectifying features of relating (i.e., looking at) in nursing while maintaining the foundational orientation to the subjectivity of the recipient of nursing care, to whom they refer as "the nursed" (Paterson & Zderad, 1978), seems to underlie this reformulation.

A noted Buber scholar (Manheim, 1974) pointed out that Buber understood that not all relationships at all times must reflect the ideal I-Thou relation. According to Manheim (1974), in some "fruit-ful" (p. 38) relationships, relations of "imbalance" are the appro-priate norm. These "unbalanced" (Manheim, 1974, p. 38) relation-ships do not contain "complete reciprocity" (p. 37). Using as examples of these unbalanced relationships the teacher-pupil and the patient-therapist relationship, Manheim (1974) suggests that a "genuine Thou relationship, for instance, can hover between teacher and pupil" (p. 38). The mutuality is incomplete because the pupil (or patient) "cannot exercise the same participation in the mutual situation, except if it were in a transfer to a friendship. . . . Buber believes that, whenever an aim is to be accomplished, mutuality cannot be complete" (Manheim, 1974, p. 38).

With regard to the outcomes of this relating, Paterson and Zderad (1988) posit that of "comfort" (p. 99). This is defined as "an um-brella concept under which all the other terms—growth, health, freedom and openness—could be sheltered" (Paterson & Zderad, 1988, p. 99). The chief dimension of relating, according to Paterson and Zderad's general theory of nursing, is presence. Presence is really what enables comfort. They state, "Through her [the nurse's] presence it is possible for other persons to be all they can be [i.e., be comfortable] in crisis situations of their worlds" (Paterson & Zderad, 1988, p. 56). Thus a relational statement between presence and comfort is proposed within the general theory of nursing.

What theoretical explanation is given to account for this pro-posed relationship? Paterson and Zderad (1988) draw an explana-tion of this relationship from existential philosophy, primarily the work of Buber and Marcel, who maintain "that it is through his [sic] relations with other men [sic] that a man [sic] becomes, that his [sic] unique individuality is actualized" (Paterson & Zderad, 1988, p. 16). Paraphrasing Buber (1965, cited in Paterson & Zderad, 1988), they state that knowledge of oneself as an individual comes through experiencing oneself as "this particular unique here-and-now person and other than that there-and-now person . . . to know myself as me is to see myself in relation to and distant from other selves" (p. 16). They conclude the discussion by posing that the possibility for "self-confirmation exists in any intersubjective sit-uation" (Paterson & Zderad, 1988, p. 16) but that availability and presence immediately precede choice, which is "a response to possibility" (p. 16) and through which people become more. There-fore the two major processes that underlie humanistic nursing are choice and presence. While these processes are separated for the purposes of discussion, in the lived nursing situation, they are inextricably interwoven. Together, they explain the proposed link between presence and comfort, which is the central tenet of the Paterson and Zderad's (1988) general theory of nursing.

5

Clinical Example

Paterson and Zderad (1978) describe the process of nursing as "quality caring based in the concept of community," which presupposes adequate knowledge and skill. They state that, from the simplest greeting of a patient to the most advanced resuscitation, nurses act as "imaginative artists" (1978) calling forth the actualities of patients by being open to the unique possibilities in the situation. This calling forth can be seen as a form of assessment and planning that takes place with the patient. The "intervention" phase is always occurring because assessment is ongoing; nonetheless, for purposes of understanding, this phase is similar to the point in which the envisioned potentials are brought forth and realized. This realization might take the form of an increased feeling of well-being, more-being, comfort, or growth. Thus "intervention" is accomplished by presence. Nurses help patients make choices from within the realities of their situations by sharing their knowledge and experience and nurturing a patient's responsible choosing. The nurse and the nursed together search for the meaning in the health-illness situation. Clinical nursing can therefore be seen as comfort promotion by means of a process of presencing.

One specific approach to comfort promotion that has been described by Zderad (1978) is the process of listening to others and living past events through with them. This allows the experience to be reinterpreted by the patient and facilitates the development of a new perspective on the experience. Zderad (1978) speaks of this process as one that deals with the effects of the past and future on the "here-and-now" (p. 68). Other specific comfort promoting strategies have been elucidated by Paterson and Zderad (1988, pp. 99-100) and have been enlivened by a detailed clinical example from psychiatric nursing in the major text (1988, pp. 113-119). Many of these aspects of humanistic nursing practice theory can be discerned in the following illustration, which comes from the writer's nursing experience within a primary health care context in an urban setting.

Example of Humanistic Nursing Practice

Jack was an African American man in his early 40s who was referred by a community health nurse to our primary nursing care practice for ongoing health care. Community health nurses staffed our hospital's walk-in referral service. Jack had made only sporadic health care visits to various medical providers across the 20-year period that followed a lengthy hospitalization in his early 20s for meningitis secondary to tuberculosis. He lived alone and was supported by a meager welfare allotment. He described a profound distrust and fear of hospitals and doctors and prided himself in a fierce independence that had enabled him to live independently despite significant memory loss related to the earlier meningitis. Nonetheless, certain symptoms would prompt Jack to seek health care.

Jack's first visit to our practice was one such occasion. His symptom of concern at the time was a cough. When listening to Jack's description of his concern, the nurse became aware of Jack's terror regarding the cough, which seemed out of proportion to the severity of the clinical picture. When Jack was invited to explore his feelings and perceptions related to the symptom, he readily revealed fear of a recurrence of tuberculosis. In addition, he was reliving his fears of being hospitalized for an extended time and held the past hospitalization of 20 years before very close to the current time. For example, he worried about disclosing the etiology of his "memory problem" to anyone for fear they would avoid him due to fears of contagion. This fear had contributed to the development of an interpersonal relating style that encouraged distance and evasion rather than friendship or intimacy. Significant losses had accompanied his prior illness experience. His wife had divorced him during the course of his lengthy hospitalization and had withheld visitation privileges of their only son. Jack's mother, who had been his major source of nurturance throughout the 20 years following his lengthy hospitalization, had recently died. Jack's ruggedly independent way of being in the world was severely threatened as he experienced frightening symptoms and tried to face them alone. Jack's call was heard by the nurse, who responded with an invitation to further dialogue.

During the first visit with Jack, the nurse focused on his concerns related to recurrence and began to explore with him the significance of the illness experience of 20 years ago. These issues were addressed by the engagement of the nurse and Jack in a presencing process that wove together the health history, physical examination, and narrative accounts of Jack's current concern and past illness experiences. Jack responded to the nurse's call to explore both his current concerns and his past illness experience; Jack's well-being was restored when his fears were acknowledged and addressed. In addition, Jack left the visit feeling hopeful about coming to a greater understanding of what he termed his "memory problem" during future planned visits to the nursing service.

Jack's hope was lived out through the experience of more-being that can be discerned in Jack's life over the next four years. During this time Jack remained a continuing client of the nursing service and maintained a primary health care relationship with the nurse with whom he had initially connected. Within this relationship across the years, limits and possibilities of living with chronic memory impairment were explored. Jack elected to participate in a vocational rehabilitation program as well as a high school equivalency program, during which he confronted the limits of his analytic ability. Never able to pass a required math class, Jack worked through a choice to disclose his past history to the instructor so that alternate learning experiences could be planned. Jack was ultimately able to secure a more stable financial status for himself by qualifying for medical disability instead of general welfare and by using his vocational skills for part-time work. He proudly reported to the nurse that he was happy now to pay for his office calls to the nursing service!

Across this four-year time period, the more-being of the nurse also grew steadily. The ongoing relationship with Jack and others within the context of an autonomous nursing group practice was the fountainhead of much learning about dependence, independence, and interdependence. This learning endures as a guiding insight for the nurse's ongoing clinical scholarship.

6

Scholarship Related to the Model

Review of the scholarship related to humanistic nursing practice theory reveals that the work is commonly cited in discussions of qualitative methods, philosophies of nursing science, ethical aspects of nursing science, and summaries of major theoretical perspectives in nursing. In addition, many researchers continue to refer to humanistic nursing practice theory and/or the process of nursology as they discuss their findings. This is particularly noted in research in the areas of caring and presence (Brown, 1986; Drew, 1986), dialogue and mutuality in relationship (Baer & Lowery, 1987; Rigdon, Clayton, & Dimond, 1987), humanism and nursing, empathy, and in research related to common existentialist themes such as loneliness (Mahon, 1982) and commitment. A few studies have used the metatheory as a guide for the study proper; only these few studies are included in the research bibliography. Thus humanistic nursing has awakened new understandings of the nursing situation and continues to inspire new ways of thinking about nursing. As a metatheory, it continues to hold promise for inviting further theoretical formulations.

7

Future Direction of Humanistic Nursing Practice Theory

Paterson and Zderad's (1988) work underscores two of the essential tensions within the nurse-patient relationship: namely, the need to balance the purely human elements of the encounter with the professional dimensions of the relationship and the related issue of boundaries within the relationship as a function of its purposiveness. The importance of this aspect of their work will continue to be recognized by scholars of the nurse-patient relationship. In addition, Paterson and Zderad's work will likely provide direction for fruitful systematic ethical inquiry.

Ethical Considerations

The nature of the nurse-patient relationship in light of its purposiveness has recently been discussed as having a critical ethical dimension in, for example, the work of Gadow (1985). Gadow states that nursing care requires "attending to the 'objectness' of persons without reducing them to the moral status of objects" (Gadow, 1985, pp. 33-34). The issue has also been discussed in the recent work of Bishop and Scudder (1990). Scudder, in earlier work with Mickunas (1985, cited in Bishop & Scudder, 1990), posits a necessary reformulation of Buber's (1953) "I-Thou" relationship when it is used to describe relations between nurses and patients. Scudder and Mickunas do so in a manner similar to that of Paterson and Zderad (1976, 1988). Scudder and Mickunas (1985, cited in Bishop & Scudder, 1990) state: "Such relationships between nurse and patient could neither be described as I-Thou or as I-It but could be described as I-It (Thou)" (p. 148). Such relationships are ones in which "a person is recognized as a person, even when limited time, the need for routine precision, or the patient care situation requires impersonal treatment" (Bishop & Scudder, 1990, p. 148). It is not known if Paterson and Zderad's (1976, 1988) work influenced Gadow or Bishop and Scudder despite the similarities with which they reformulated Buber's thought for use in nursing relationships. Gadow's work and its similarity to their own work is pointed out by Bishop and Scudder (1990, pp. 154, 156). These independent working styles typify the lack of connectedness among nurse ethicists and nurse theorists in the area of the nurse-patient relationship as well as in other domains of inquiry within nursing (Reed, 1989; Sarter, 1988). As the ethical nature of theorizing is increasingly realized in nursing (Reed, 1989; Yeo, 1989), Paterson and Zderad's humanistic nursing practice theory will be recognized for its strengths in this regard and for its consonance with the ethical positions put forward by Gadow (1985) and Bishop and Scudder (1990).

Current Resources

Because Paterson and Zderad are both retired from nursing, it seems particularly important to include the names of scholars who are currently engaged in work arising from humanistic nursing practice theory. Paterson and Zderad (personal communication, July, 1991) identify several people as being currently engaged in such work: (a) Dr. Sumiko Fujiki, 600 New Stine Road, Apt. 22, Bakersfield, CA 93309-2970 (psychiatric mental health nursing educator); telephone: 805-664-3111 (work) and 805-397-1699 (home). (b) Doris R. Hines, Ph.D., R.N., RR#1, Box 341, Agency, MS 64401; telephone: 816-271-7111 (page through operator), 816-271-7707 (office) 816-253-9443 (home) (clinical nurse specialist in adult health and researcher). Those listed here have expressed their willingness to serve as resources for future development of humanistic nursing practice theory.

In addition, the writer is interested in applications of humanistic nursing practice theory in nonpsychiatric nursing settings, in particular in adult primary health care contexts. She can be reached at Oakland University School of Nursing, Rochester, MI 49309-4401; telephone: 313-370-4076 (office) and 313-549-6398 (home).

Glossary

All-at-once.
"Awareness of living many concepts, emotions, desires, values in a particular instance dispels narrow singularity of purpose and complements wisdom" (Paterson, 1978, p. 51).

Between.
Mutual presence of the nurse-nursed; "the basic relation in which and through which nursing can occur" (Paterson & Zderad, 1988, p. 22); the realm of intersubjective experience.

Choice.
"Response to possibility" (Paterson & Zderad, 1988, p. 16).

Clinical.
"Aware presence in the health situation" (Paterson, 1978, p. 51).

Comfort.
"Persons being all they can be in particular life situations" (Paterson, 1978, p. 51).

Complementary synthesis.
Seeing through multiple realities to a unified insight.

Empathy.
"Imaginative moving towards oneness with another, sharing his [or her] being in a situation, resulting in an insightful knowledge of his [or her] perspective" (Paterson, 1978, p. 51).

44

More-being.
The *becoming* aspect of the being-becoming polarity.

Multifarious multiplicities.
The complex nature of the nursing situation with its diverse concerns.

Noetic locus.
Source of knowing; refers to the synthesis of knowledge that occurs within humans.

Nursology.
Phenomenological method of inquiry into nursing phenomena aimed toward developing nursing theory.

Nurturance.
"Promoting growth through relating" (Paterson, 1978, p. 51).

Phenomenology.
A descriptive method of inquiry into the nature of phenomena *as experienced.*

Presence.
"Being with" another as compared with "seeming-to-be"; existential relating of one being-as-being to another being-as-being.

Transaction.
A descriptor highlighting the two-way nature of relating; the relating goes both ways between participants.

Well-being.
The being aspect of the being-becoming polarity.

References

American Nurses' Association (ANA). (1980). *Nursing: A social policy statement.* Kansas City, MO: Author.

Baer, E. D., & Lowery, B. J. (1987). Patient and situational factors that affect nursing students' like or dislike of caring for patients. *Nursing Research, 36*(5), 298-302.

Benner, P., & Wrubel, J. (1989). *The primacy of caring.* New York: Addison-Wesley.

Bishop, A. H., & Scudder, J. R. (1990). *The practical, moral, and personal sense of nursing: A phenomenological philosophy of practice.* Albany: State University of New York Press.

Brown, L. (1986). The experience of care: Patient perspectives. *Topics in Clinical Nursing, 8*(2), 56-62.

Buber, M. (1953). I and Thou. In W. Herberg (Ed.), *The writings of Martin Buber* (pp. 43-62). New York: World.

Drew, M. (1986). Exclusion and confirmation: A phenomenology of patient's experiences with caregivers. *Image: Journal of Nursing Scholarship, 18*(2), 39-43.

Fawcett, J. (1980). A framework for analysis and evaluation of conceptual models. *Nurse Educator, 5*(6), 10-14.

Fawcett, J. (1984). *Analysis and evaluation of conceptual models of nursing.* Philadelphia: F. A. Davis.

Flaskerud, J. H., & Halloran, E. J. (1980). Areas of agreement in nursing theory. *Advances in Nursing Science, 3*(1), 1-7.

Gadow, S. A. (1985). Nurse and patient: The caring relationship. In A. H. Bishop & J. Scudder (Eds.), *Caring, curing, coping* (pp. 31-43). University, AL: University of Alabama Press.

Guigan, C. (1986). Existentialist ethics. In J. P. Demarco & R. M. Fox (Eds.), *New directions in ethics* (pp. 73-91). New York: Routledge & Kegan Paul.

Leininger, M. M. (1985). *Qualitative research methods in nursing*. Orlando, FL: Grune & Stratton.

Mahon, N. E. (1982). The relationship of self-disclosure, interpersonal dependency, and life changes to loneliness in young adults. *Nursing Research, 31*(6), 343-347.

Manheim, W. (1974). *Martin Buber*. New York: Twayne.

Newman, M. A. (1983). The continuing revolution: A history of nursing science. In N. L. Chaska (Ed.), *The nursing profession: A time to speak* (pp. 385-393). New York: McGraw-Hill.

Parse, R. R. (1987). *Nursing science: Major paradigms, theories and critiques*. Philadelphia: W. B. Saunders.

Paterson, J. G. (1971). From a philosophy of clinical nursing to a method of nursology. *Nursing Research, 20*(2), 143-146.

Paterson, J. G. (1978). The tortuous way toward nursing theory. In *Theory development: What, why, how?* (NLN Publ. No. 15-1708, pp. 49-65). New York: National League for Nursing.

Paterson, J. G., & Zderad, L. T. (1976). *Humanistic nursing*. New York: John Wiley.

Paterson, J. G., & Zderad, L. T. (Speakers). (1978). *Humanistic nursing practice theory* (Audio cassette). From the Second Annual Nurse Educator Conference, New York. New York: Concept Media.

Paterson, J. G., & Zderad, L. T. (1988). *Humanistic nursing* (NLN Publ. No. 41-2218; 2nd ed.). New York: National League for Nursing.

Reed, P. G. (1989). Nursing theorizing as an ethical endeavor. *Advances in Nursing Science, 11*(3), 1-9.

Rigdon, I. S., Clayton, B. C., & Dimond, M. (1987). Toward a theory of helpfulness for the elderly bereaved: An invitation to a new life. *Advances in Nursing Science, 9*(2), 32-43.

Sarter, B. (1988). Philosophical sources of nursing theory. *Nursing Science Quarterly, 1*, 52-59.

Smith, J. A. (1981). The idea of health: A philosophic inquiry. *Advances in Nursing Science, 3*(3), 43-50.

Stevens, B. J. (1990). *Nursing theory analysis, application, evaluation* (3rd ed.). Glenview, IL: Scott Foresman/Little, Brown.

White, M. (1983). *The age of analysis*. Boston: Houghton Mifflin.

Yeo, M. (1989). Integration of nursing theory and nursing ethics. *Advances in Nursing Science, 11*(3), 33-43.

Zbilut, J. P. (1980). Holistic nursing: The transcendental factor. *Nursing Forum, 19*(1), 45-49.

Zderad, L. T. (1969). Empathic nursing: Realization of a human capacity. *Nursing Clinics of North America, 4*, 655-662.

Zderad, L. T. (1978). From here and now to theory: Reflections on "how." *Theory development: What, why, how?* (NLN Publ. No. 15-1708, pp. 35-48). New York: National League for Nursing.

Bibliography

Published Works of Paterson and Zderad

Paterson, J. G. (1971). From a philosophy of clinical nursing to a method of nursology. *Nursing Research, 20*(2), 143-146.

Paterson, J. G. (1978). The tortuous way toward nursing theory. In *Theory development: What, why, how?* (NLN Publ. No. 15-1708, pp. 49-65). New York: National League for Nursing.

Paterson, J. G., & Zderad, L. T. (1970). *All together through complementary syntheses the worlds of the many. Image, 4*(3), 13-16.

Paterson, J. G., & Zderad, L. T. (1976). *Humanistic nursing.* New York: John Wiley.

Paterson, J. G., & Zderad, L. T. (1988). *Humanistic nursing* (NLN Publ. No. 41-2218). New York: National League for Nursing.

Zderad, L. T. (1969). Empathic nursing: Realization of a human capacity. *Nursing Clinics of North America, 4,* 655-662.

Zderad, L. T. (1970). Empathy: From cliché to construct. In *Proceedings of the Third Nursing Theory Conference* (pp. 46-75). Lawrence: University of Kansas Medical Center, Department of Nursing.

Zderad, L. T. (1978). From here and now to theory: Reflections on "how." *Theory development: What, why, how?* (NLN Publ. No. 15-1708, pp. 35-48). New York: National League for Nursing.

Summary, Critique, and Analysis

Brouse, S. H., & Laffrey, S. C. (1989). Paterson & Zderad's humanistic nursing framework. In J. J. Fitzpatrick & A. H. Whall (Eds.), *Conceptual models of nursing: Analysis and application* (pp. 205-225). (2nd ed.). Norwalk, CT: Appleton-Lange.

Kleinman, S. (1986). Humanistic nursing: The phenomenological theory of Paterson & Zderad. In P. Winstead-Fry (Ed.), *Case studies in nursing theory* (NLN Publ. No. 15-2152, pp. 167-195). New York: National League for Nursing.

Meleis, A. F. (1991). *Theoretical nursing: Development and progress*. New York: Lippincott.

Praeger, S. G., & Hogarth, C. R. (1990). Josephine E. Paterson and Loretta T. Zderad. In J. B. George (Ed.), *Nursing theories: The base for professional practice* (pp. 287-299). (3rd ed.). Norwalk, CT: Appleton-Lange.

Stevens, B. J. (1990). *Nursing theory analysis, application, evaluation* (3rd ed.). Glenview, IL: Scott Foresman/Little, Brown.

General Commentary

Boyd, C. O. (1990). Critical appraisal of developing nursing research methods. *Nursing Science Quarterly, 3*(1), 42-43.

Cohen, M. Z. (1987). A historical overview of the phenomenologic movement. *Image: Journal of Nursing Scholarship, 19*(1), 31-34.

Munhall, P. L., & Oiler, C. J. (1986). *Nursing research: A qualitative perspective*. Norwalk, CT: Appleton-Century-Crofts.

Oiler, C. J. (1986). Qualitative methods: Phenomenology. In P. Moccia (Ed.), *New approaches to theory development* (NLN Publ. No. 15-1992, pp. 75-103). New York: National League for Nursing.

Sarter, B. (1987). Evolutionary idealism: A philosophical foundation for holistic nursing theory. *Advances in Nursing Science, 9*(2), 1-9.

Taylor, S. G. (1985). Rights and responsibilities: Nurse-patient relationships. *Image: Journal of Nursing Scholarship, 17*(1), 9-13.

Watson, J. (1981). Nursing's scientific quest. *Nursing Outlook, 29,* 413-416.

Research

Hinds, P. S. (1988). The relationship of nurses' caring behaviors with hopefulness and health care outcomes in adolescents. *Archives of Psychiatric Nursing, 2*(1), 21-29.

Hines, D. R. (1991). *The development of the measurement of presence scale*. Unpublished doctoral dissertation, Texas Woman's University.

Kleinman, S. (1986). Humanistic nursing: The phenomenological theory of Paterson & Zderad. In P. Winstead-Fry (Ed.), *Case studies in nursing theory* (NLN Publ. No. 15-2152, pp. 167-195). New York: National League for Nursing.

Pettigrew, J. M. (1988). *A phenomenological study of the nurse's presence with persons experiencing suffering*. Unpublished doctoral dissertation, Texas Woman's University.

About the Author

Nancy O'Connor (R.N., C. M.S.N.) is Assistant Professor of Nursing at Oakland University in Rochester, Michigan. She is also certified by the American Nurses' Association as an Adult Nurse Practitioner. She is currently a doctoral student in nursing at Wayne State University in Detroit, Michigan. Her research interests include the nurse-patient relationship, primary care nursing practice, and nursing education for advanced clinical practice.